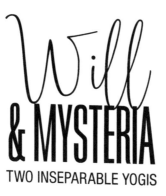

Will & MYSTERIA

TWO INSEPARABLE YOGIS

CHRISTA REYNOLDS

◆ FriesenPress

Suite 300 - 990 Fort St
Victoria, BC, V8V 3K2
Canada

www.friesenpress.com

Copyright © 2019 by Christa Reynolds
First Edition — 2019

Will & Mysteria is available at special quantity discounts for bulk purchase for sales promotion, fund-raising, speaking engagements and educational needs. Special workbooks and materials can be provided for educational programs. For details write christa.reynolds@comcast.net

ISBN
978-1-5255-4552-8 (Hardcover)
978-1-5255-4553-5 (Paperback)
978-1-5255-4554-2 (eBook)

1. HEALTH & FITNESS, YOGA

Distributed to the trade by The Ingram Book Company

"*Will & Mysteria* is a beautiful allegory of self awareness and inner thought. It's a potent and timeless tale of the struggle to stay true to your inner truth and intuition amongst the strong call of one's ego and desire for success. I have found myself re-reading it and uncovering more wisdom with each read. Its a book to be shared and referenced...appropriate for everyone of all ages."
Denise Dresser, SVP
Technology Executive, Salesforce

"I once told Christa Reynolds that I tried to perform random acts of kindness. To which she replied, "Why random? Why not do it every day?" *Will & Mysteria* is about "doing it every day.""
Richard Polsky, author
I bought Andy Warhol

"Love your book! Just like your photography, your book is an illustration of the beauty of being oneself."
Romy David
Spirit Rock Meditation Coordinator

"A lovely and imaginative book, an easy blend of physical and mental, spiritual, and secular, with (best of all) exercises to be practiced."
Rev. Hosho Peter Coyote, Zen Buddhist priest.

"A modern day Icarus with an internal twist"
Mary Sherman
Hanson Bridgett

With Great Love...

I'm dedicating Will and Mysteria to my father, who passed when I was 18 years old, and nudges me along in dreamtime, to my mother who inspired my creativity, to my long-term yoga students who have believed in me and have supported me with their beautiful wisdom and to everyone out there who desires to be free and in magical alignment with their inner world!

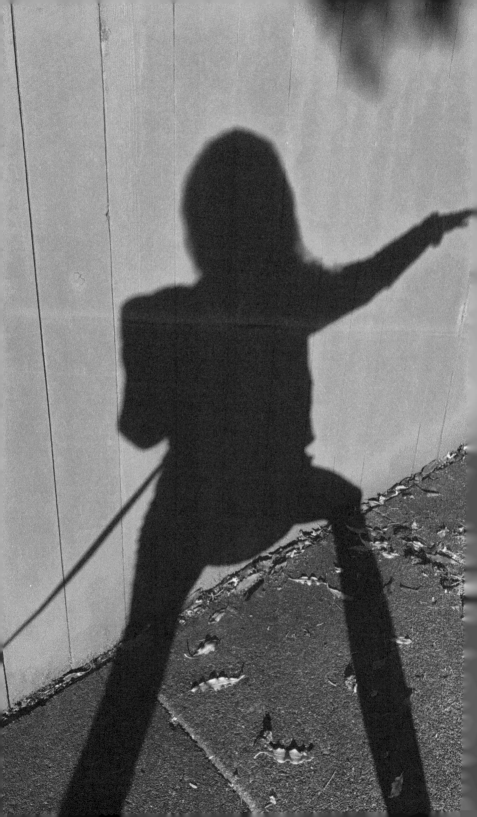

INTRODUCTION

Yoga is mythic. It's our divine union with the sun and the moon, the yin and the yang. It's our inhale in relationship to our exhale. When practiced with presence, it supports us, transcending the current gender gap, the external as well as the internal judgments we find ourselves wading through, and this limited dimension we're just beginning to discard. We're unfolding each moment either by adding or subtracting "story" to our personal myth. We are students of yoga continuously learning as we go, opening constantly to wonderment, unpacking challenges as they arise, or cleaning up after each unconscious blunder.

It's my invitation to you as you read this myth/modern day parable to take a Will and Mysteria moment each time you see (WM) show up in the story. Will and Mysteria will reveal themselves early on in the story, indicating their power and preciousness. Reflect on their existence, their sound, and your feelings while observing your mind's relationship to them. I hope you enjoy this story and end up reading it a few times, for there are hidden gems throughout.

Much love,
    Christa

I n the abundant and plentiful province of Galore, a coastal wonderland, there lived two inseparable friends named Will and Mysteria. These two distinct energies resided deep within the bodily framework of a young man named Oliver Humane. Will and Mysteria were responsible for Oliver's internal movements, his life force traveling through his body, his basic temperament, and his connection to life itself. They shared complementary purposes; neither could exist without the other, nor could Oliver exist without them. As Will and Mysteria became more and more present in Oliver's awareness, they found themselves to be quite invaluable.

Oliver was awed by their insistent and yet subtle ability to get his attention, guiding him toward peacefulness and consciousness. As you'll see over the course of this story and Oliver's travails, he began to comprehend Will and

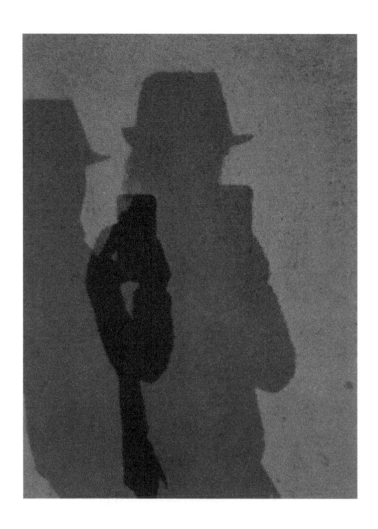

Mysteria's true natures, their ability to expand and contract, excite or calm, connect feelings with awareness and consciousness. Although Oliver had hardly known they existed most of his life, this would all begin to change when he'd have to override his internal urges and depend on them for his life's entertainment and companionship.

* * *

Oliver, a young, ambitious engineer and professor at Galore University, was filled with an innovative spirit and a desire to prove his convictions. He enjoyed experimenting with industrial designs and the law of gravity. When Oliver was not at the university, he could be found on coastal cliffs and tall buildings measuring the velocity of falling objects. He would play with coins and feathers, observing their movement and flow patterns. Oliver thrived on innovation and felt a great need to make a difference in the world.

What drove this ambition? Besides having a curious and brilliant mind, Oliver was the middle child in a family of five children, and he had an enormous desire to excel—to be noticed. Oliver found early on in his life how easy it was to disappear within the chatter of his crowded family. In the rare moments when he was

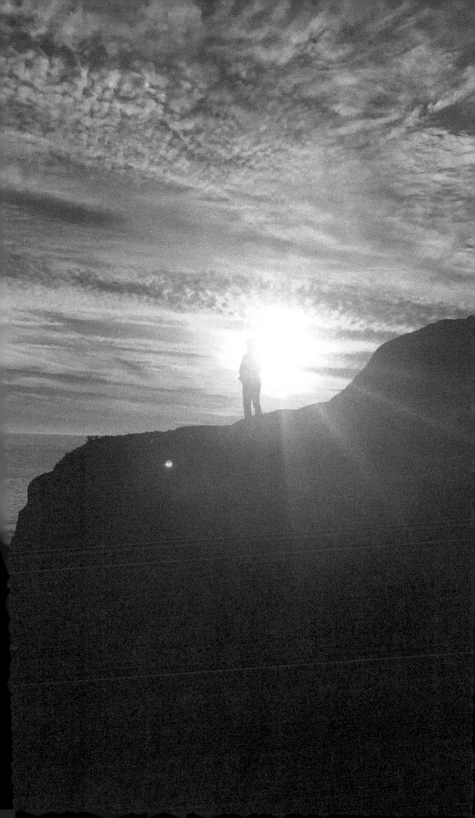

showered with adulation and appreciation, his whole being lit up, and his heart opened. He was motivated by the need to be seen, to feel loved, and to give his love back to the world.

Oliver's parents, Harold and Judith, were greatly respected by the people of Galore for their humanitarian efforts, caring for the community's orphaned children and teens. Harold and Judith felt that youth by their very nature needed both male and female role models to guide them through life, and they devoted themselves to being those guardians for many of the town's orphans. As a result, however, Harold and Judith were often so busy attending to everyone else's needs they became unaware of their own children's needs, often leaving the young Humanes to fend for themselves while growing up.

Fortunately for Oliver, the province of Galore was lush with vegetation, vast coastal cliffs, a vibrant economy, and ample opportunities for growth and expansion. This presented the perfect setting for his innovations and creativity to unfold. It was often said by the many who visited this glorious coastal town that "those who resided in the land of Galore had everything they ever needed and more."

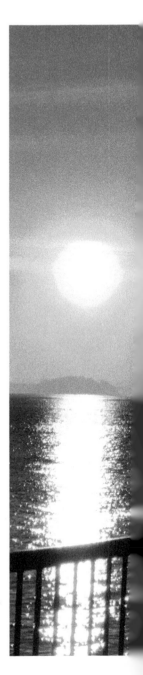

Will and Mysteria having their own consciousness were thrilled to be Oliver's respiration—his internal world of expansive inhales and liberated exhales. They shared an essential job and a yoga practice he was only beginning to become aware of. **When you see (WM) throughout the story, it's a reminder to pause and take a slow deep inhale and a softening and relaxing exhale.**

Will's job was to fill Oliver with life itself, expanding his presence from the inside as he naturally drew oxygen inward through his lungs, becoming energized and powerful. (WM) This physical initiative fed his body with inspiration and a spirit so vital and joyful it was infectious. Others could bask in this exuberance and reflect its warrior-like nature and vibrancy. Will could draw from his environment the most exciting energy and fill Oliver with purpose and pure radiance. This sun-sourced energy imbued Oliver with a feeling of trust for his environment, an ambitious wherewithal for his inspirations, and an instinctual excitement for life itself. (WM)

Mysteria, in contrast, appeared and disappeared with great alacrity. Her innate ability to surrender and let go, releasing muscle tension from the lungs and the rest of the body, often united her with profound truths. (WM) She traveled deep and penetrated the complexity of the unconscious and cell structure of Oliver's mind and body. Encouraged by Will's light, she could dislodge old cellular memory, freeing Oliver's cells for present-time information. (WM) She sensed life on its own terms; she enjoyed new things but approached them with inquiry and caution. Her intelligence would often alert her that

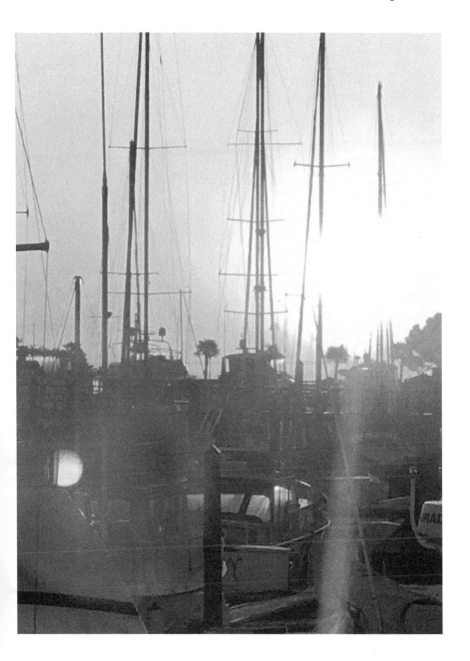

all things were not what they seemed in the reflection of the moon's light. (WM)

Will's expansive brightness, which made him game for everything, and Mysteria's great ability to release and surrender, even in the face of great unknowns, complemented each other beautifully, making them a wonderful team within Oliver Humane. (WM)

Just as Will and Mysteria would begin to find their rhythm within Oliver's well-conditioned body, another indweller named Edgar would rear his indulgent spirit. Edgar resided primarily in Oliver's mind and was always planning for the future or rehashing past events. Edgar's hypervigilance to stay busy and in the limelight left Oliver very little time to really connect with anybody, especially Will and Mysteria. As a result, Edgar often complicated life within Oliver for Will and Mysteria. Left to their own natures, they maneuvered in a balanced manner, but Edgar "being Edgar-possessed", liked to overshadow them. (WM) His charming personality gave the mistaken impression that he actually cared about the others living in Oliver. Edgar was both seductive and clever, coercing others to follow his spectacular agenda— all of which made him appealing and caused Will and Mysteria to virtually disappear for what felt like minutes or even hours at a time. He was always looking for an angle, following the next money-making idea, or trying to uphold his inflated reputation. (WM)

Why did Will and Mysteria even bother to pay attention to Edgar and work with him? Well, for one reason, Edgar prompted many of Oliver's attitudes and

behaviors. For another, they had been neighbors within Oliver's body from time eternal. Edgar was often the only connection Will and Mysteria had to Oliver's mind. And mere proximity kept them mixed up in one another's lives. (WM)

Despite their different approaches to life, Will and Mysteria found Edgar entertaining and appreciated many of his clever ideas. Still, they continually tried to quiet Edgar's forced intellect, his need to be right, and his many contradictions. Edgar worked diligently to exude confidence and power, but he had to work equally hard to conceal Oliver's fears, vulnerabilities, and shortcomings. (WM) With his rapid defensive nature "the truth" often eluded him. Once, he encouraged Oliver to sound off in the local newspaper about Galore's need to recycle and "go green." Days later, Oliver was observed dropping cans and bottles into the town square trash basket. This unconscious blunder had the editorial staff all too eager to point out Oliver's laziness and hypocrisy. (WM)

As the seasons changed, so did life inside Oliver for Will and Mysteria. With spring approaching, Oliver, who had always been interested in gravitational studies was finding himself driven by an aspiration to fly. The desire had come to him after Edgar showed him how to build a set of wings made of strong, intricate hawk feathers.

"Listen," Edgar urged, "these wings will catch the thermals of any crosswind and lift your body to great heights. There's nothing like them."

Edgar's ambitions inspired Will—after all, he was easily excited, sometimes gasping with fright but mostly game for anything. Mysteria, on the other hand, was immediately skeptical. "Hang on a minute," she said. "We are part of the human condition. We don't fly; we steward the earth!" she exclaimed. (WM)

But Will's enthusiasm was as bright as the lights on a Christmas tree. He could not imagine letting this opportunity pass by. He recalled the many times Oliver had dreamed of flying, ascending from the earth's surface, rising above everything. Will began to envision himself soaring in line with the sun and all its brilliant energy. His interest was innocent, even naive, but the sheer idea made him ecstatic.

Edgar kept up his persuasion. "Flying with hawk-feather wings is a courageous act, one nobody has tried recently or ever been successful at."

Then, after unconsciously skipping over a much-needed Will and Mysteria moment, Edgar blurted out to Will, "This ability will separate Oliver from everyone else. He'll be famous! He'll be able to manufacture millions of these wings and sell them to everyone. He'll be rich and powerful."

Mysteria immediately set about inspecting the wings for safety and craftsmanship. She felt an imminent danger, yet she didn't want to quash Oliver's dreams. Even though everything about the wings appeared to be in working order, she shuddered as she exhaled in fearful frustration. (WM) "Will, I don't believe we should try this risky undertaking. Has anyone else tried these wings to make sure they are durable and capable of taking a human into flight?" she asked.

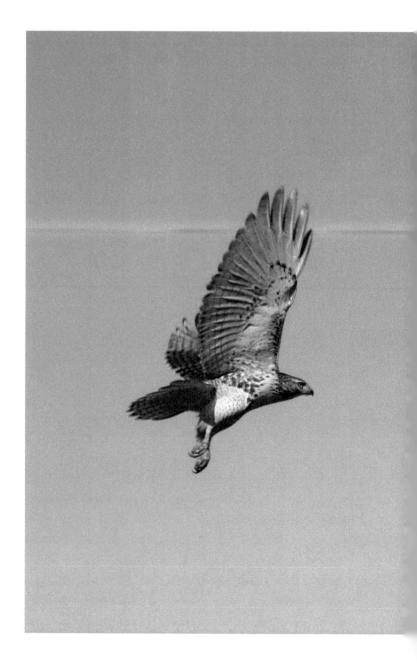

Will replied reluctantly, "Well, no. We will be the first."

"Oliver Humane will change the world as we know it!" Edgar crowed.

Mysteria was aroused by Will and Edgar's excitement. Still, she wondered why they had to be the ones to change the world on such a grand scale. "Could we attain this exalted state by trying to meditate and levitate instead? Maybe we can fly this way first?" she asked. (WM)

"That's been done by the yogis in India," said Edgar dismissively. "Now it's time to take real flight and show the world that Oliver Humane can rise above the mundane and soar."

"But we need the mundane," Mysteria explained. "We need the earth and its materials to survive. We are not above them." (WM)

Will listened intently to both sides and acknowledged the value in both perspectives. His inhalation quickened as Mysteria's exhalation was released with greater agitation. (WM) Meanwhile, Edgar's scheming mind was shifting quickly with excitement.

* * *

That evening, Will and Mysteria were curt with each other as they tried to fall asleep, anticipating the next day's adventure. Instead of the good night's sleep they needed, they spent a long night wrestling with Edgar's shadow. They kept getting pulled into a disturbing dream

Oliver was having, in which his parents arrived late to the air show and missed his whole flight. (WM)

Will and Mysteria woke the next morning agitated, knowing that their fate, and Oliver's, hung in the balance that day. Looking out the window at a dark, overcast day, they wondered why the birds were not chirping. (WM) They felt a sense of dread mixed with excitement, which gradually morphed into a light-headed state. (WM)

Edgar greeted them by saying, "This is the day Oliver Humane will revolutionize human transportation. Journalists and photographers will capture our miraculous feat. It will be amazing, and he will be responsible."

A vision suddenly came to Mysteria and she exclaimed, "What if we crash? What if the wings fail us?" (WM)

Will again found himself caught between these two viewpoints. He could understand Mysteria's concern, but the exhilaration and future adulation were far more appealing to concentrate on.

Mysteria tried to be diplomatic. "I see the beauty in what we're trying to accomplish, Will. There's real freedom in flying. It's miraculous! I want to support you in this endeavor, and yet I have a feeling we are in danger." (WM)

At Edgar's insistence, Will then proclaimed, "The world needs this accomplishment. Each moment of every day someone somewhere in the world risks his life so that we as a species might progress to the next level of evolution. I won't let anything happen to us, Mysteria." Will trembled through these last words.

Mysteria emitted a long sigh, prompting Edgar to blurt out, "You can't keep worrying, Mysteria. This is Oliver's moment. He will be nothing without this flight."

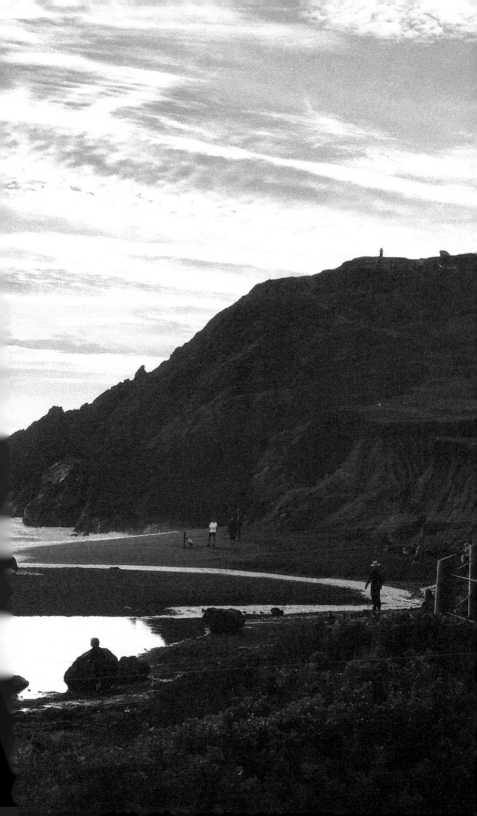

Upon the release of her being (WM), she murmured, "Or he might become nothing by trying these wings."

Mysteria then began to do what she's inherently inclined to do: let go. (WM) She hoped someday this would all make sense even though it didn't at that moment. She gathered her strength, readying herself for the flight ahead. She and Will worked together to find a rhythm as they tried to calm Oliver's central nervous system for the challenge ahead. (WM)

People from all over Galore had congregated at the beach to see the momentous event. Oliver, with all his internal inhabitants, began climbing to the mid-level cliff some thirty feet above the spectators of Galore. He carried the hawk-feather wings himself, showing the crowd how light they were. Edgar had chosen to launch from this specific cliff height so it would lift Oliver into flight right away and show the people of Galore how easily the thermals carried him upward. As he donned the wings, they all paused for a long moment. The vibration of fear running through Oliver was palpable, his knees were shaking and his heart pounding. Will and Mysteria all but disappeared, getting lost in Edgar's fears, only to be suddenly coughed back into existence. (WM) They quickly resumed their positions and began to assure each other of their great love and friendship. Will told Mysteria, "Even if we must give our last breath for this adventure, I will gladly join you on the other side." Mysteria exhaled with great relief. They both knew at that moment they had nothing to lose, no matter how the journey turned out. (WM)

Edgar, on the other hand, was nauseated listening to their devotional exchange, realizing the magnitude of the task before Oliver. (WM) He also noticed at that moment how alone he felt. He found himself desperately searching for Oliver's parents below. He needed reassurance. Upon seeing Harold and Judith in the crowd, a mild relief began to creep in, but then the spectators' enthusiasm and cheers escalated him back into worry.

"What have I gotten us into?" Edgar asked himself quietly. Out loud, Oliver nervously said, "I need to get this show going." Edgar then impatiently gave Oliver a quick nudge, launching him off the cliff. Falling prey to a great moment of panic, he disappeared into a deep unconscious state—almost entirely missing the flight. As Oliver took flight, Will and Mysteria were lifted immediately by the warm ocean thermals under the beautiful hawk feathers. Like a steep drop on a roller coaster, this gust of air took away their purpose momentarily.

Then, suddenly lifted, they were astounded by the height and speed at which the wings ascended them into the stormy-looking skies. They realized they were in fact flying and could hear a long *"Wowwwww"* from the crowd below. It was exhilarating! Just then, the dark clouds divided, and the sun broke through with a glistening glow. Oliver began to rotate the wings, and they soared downward toward the crowd, finding the next heat thermal to glide through.

They turned, they twisted, and they glided. The freedom they experienced was unparalleled. They felt invincible, as if they had finally found the right perspective to everything. They spontaneously decided to wake

Edgar out of his unconscious slumber so he too could enjoy the journey. As they nudged him awake, terror filled his essence, and Oliver's body went rigid.

Suddenly, a great gust of wind kicked up and blew them off course. They desperately tried to direct their flight pattern back toward the crowd, but the wings would not cooperate with their adjustments, and the sun was all but disappearing again behind the dark clouds. Mysteria was sure she knew what terrible fate awaited them; it was just as her previous intuition and vision had warned her. Feathers began to tear off the wings as the winds were now blowing from two directions. Will and Mysteria gazed downward and realized they had flown far out to sea; all they could see was the ocean below and the coast of Galore far off in the distance.

They were out of control. Will and Mysteria realized Oliver's body had reached a height of nearly three hundred feet, when the two wings collapsed in on each other. The collapse sent them spiraling downward. Will and Mysteria felt the weight of Oliver's body as it plunged violently toward the mouth of Mother Ocean. They wanted desperately to help Oliver survive this fall. After all, he had housed their existence since his birth. It seemed, however, that Will and Mysteria's life force might not be enough to save Oliver from this deadly spiral. (WM)

In a state of quickening descent, Oliver's life was now flashing before his eyes. He began to recall the various driving forces and moments of his life: his insistent need to feel seen; his relentless need to be someone special so he could be loved and respected by his family; the many times his younger sisters had simply wanted him to read them a book, and he had been too involved in his own pursuits; the countless times his folks had asked him to join the various outings with the parentless children of Galore, and he had felt put upon and then often isolated. He was terrified, desperate for a chance to fix his mistakes, and he felt his life force leaving.

With this flight, Oliver had hoped he would finally win the attention and respect he had always thought he needed. Although his parents were petrified for their son's safety, they could not have been prouder, and they'd encouraged the whole town to come and watch.

Then, out of nowhere, Edgar reappeared—frantically, desperately pleading for another chance as Oliver's body descended rapidly. "Dear God, please help me. Please, I'll do anything ... I'll be more—"

Suddenly, a flash of bright light appeared, and all went black. (WM)

* * *

During Oliver's horrific downward spiral, both Will and Mysteria felt themselves being drawn away from his plunging body. (WM) As Oliver's physical form descended, a tremendous magnetic force lifted Will and Mysteria up and beyond the stratosphere. They traveled through warm thermals and cool air spots as they found themselves moving faster, gaining speed from this magnetic force. They noticed the earth

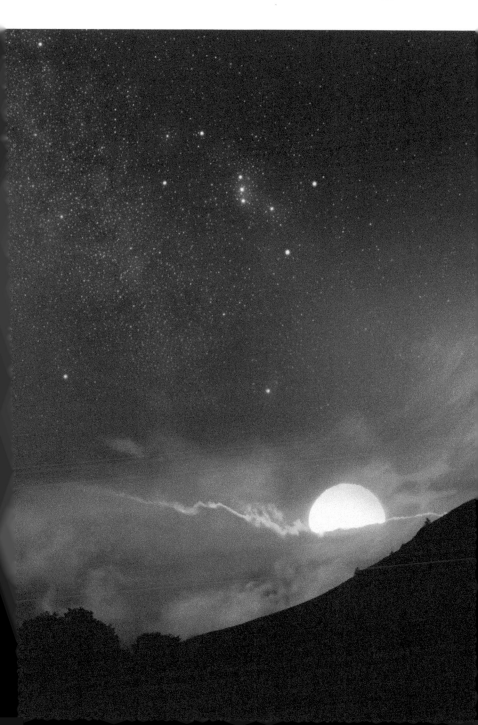

becoming smaller as the moon and sun began to reflect each other with spectacular colors. They were pulled briskly through a blinding but luminous portal and descended softly, landing on a clear crystal altar. They stayed close together as they quivered in anticipation of what lay ahead. Moments later, Edgar tumbled in, disheveled, disoriented, and dismayed by his journey. Clearly, he had traveled a different route.

They waited for what seemed like lifetimes, until they sensed a radiant energy and the crystal altar began to vibrate. The energy was so intense, they struggled to stay in their respective spots. This omnipotent force increased their vibrations to such an escalated degree they thought they might explode. Then, with a sudden blue-green flash, a stunning presence appeared, so striking, radiant, and strong it robbed them of any thought or gesture. They felt vacuous, spacey, and then completely calm. (WM)

Through this all-encompassing peaceful feeling, they soon realized it was RaLuna, the perfect mixture of the sun and the moon, the male and the female, the vision of totality and unmistakable wholeness. Both Will and Mysteria could not believe their good fortune, for RaLuna was only known to them through rare innate mystical feelings as well as the many books that Oliver had read revealing this exquisite source of energy. (WM) Edgar, however, looked uneasy and tried to shrink from RaLuna's sight.

"Wow, that's RaLuna, the universal gatekeeper for the earth's inhabitants," whispered Mysteria to Edgar and Will. "RaLuna represents the voice of the universe's almighty Source, or God.

"This is amazing! This must be about Oliver's body and our role in his survival," suggested Will. (WM)

After a moment of intense energy surges, RaLuna began by acknowledging the precariousness of their earthly journey. "You are all to be commended for your sheer faith in the earth's daily unknowns. It's an intricate and profound path you each travel. Although you reside in Oliver's physical form, it's your individual spirits that will be reviewed here today." RaLuna took a long pause. (WM)

Looking directly at Will and Mysteria, RaLuna said, "I thought you both had a handle on Edgar. I never believed that you, Will, and you, Mysteria, could still be so manipulated by Oliver's ego and all its crazy antics to make him famous and, most of all, special and separate. These repetitive feelings within Oliver are his way of staying unconscious and falsely safe. (WM) Will and Mysteria, you are life force itself, the connective source to everything. You both have an enormous ability and responsibility to help Oliver become more present, peaceful, and loving. You know Edgar is mostly concerned with Edgar."

Edgar suddenly appeared, squirming as he objected softly, "Not always."

RaLuna continued, "Yet you still give him so much power. Will, I love your enthusiasm, your expansiveness, and your desire to experience all of life. Mysteria, I commend your offerings and insights along the way; they give room for pause. (WM) Will, you need to listen more to your intuition, your feminine side. What will it take for you to recognize Edgar's real motives? He is your nemesis. (WM) Will and Mysteria, you are each whole and complete when in relation to each other. You have the power to elevate and release anything in your pathway. Your force is more powerful than can even be imagined. (WM) Conserve this energy and use it wisely, for you are made in the likeness of the Source itself. With presence and love you can manifest anything that needs to happen."

Will and Mysteria looked at each other, speechless. (WM) RaLuna continued, "You two are so easily influenced by what Oliver thinks he needs in order to be loved or to survive his social environment. In these moments, both of you need to slow down enough to exercise your precious resource to give Edgar the space to recognize and reconnect with his essential self. (WM) Your precious gifts of expansion and surrender will calm Edgar so he can use his cleverness to help the world with its real problems."

Edgar was energized by hearing RaLuna acknowledge one of his strengths. (WM)

"Edgar," exclaimed RaLuna, "your desire to excel in the world is commendable, however doing it alone is devastating for you. It ignites your inner emptiness, which causes you to grasp for anything as you try to soothe and fill in these inner reservoirs with tiring outside adventures. Fear settles in because there is no inner foundation or connection to something beyond your thoughts. This projected busyness, which feels dubiously stable as it masked the emptiness, will need to be acknowledged and transformed."

"Emptiness, really? What does RaLuna mean by this?" groaned Edgar.

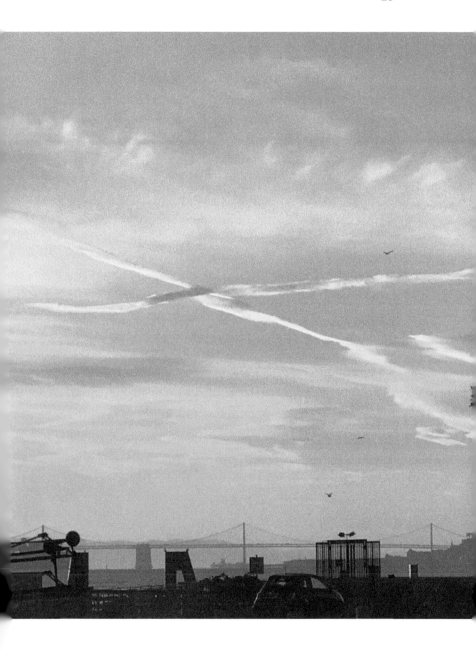

RaLuna then took a moment to evaluate Oliver's impending death, weighing whether he merited a revival and a return to earth to continue his life. (WM) Suddenly, there he was on the full-life viewer screen, frozen in midair and seconds away from crashing into the ocean's surface. RaLuna continued, "I can breathe you all back into Oliver's body, but only if you promise to take what has happened here and bring it to consciousness within him. Oliver has some major lessons ahead. Can you all be there for him, for this essential job?" (WM)

Will and Mysteria were still in awe and felt quite honored and challenged by this proposition. (WM) They looked at each other and promised to do as RaLuna asked. Edgar, on the other hand, was squirming to find a way out of there. He could feel an impending doom; he didn't see how this could end well for him. RaLuna then looked sideways at him. "You're all in this together," RaLuna announced, and he sheepishly conceded.

RaLuna's energy brightened, indicating pleasure with their decision to return. "I believe that after this transformation, Oliver will come to cherish all of you more and realize your influence and your love," exclaimed RaLuna.

With that, RaLuna breathed Will, Mysteria, and Edgar back into Oliver's body, as it continued its downward spiral. With their renewed presence, the wings began repairing themselves, slowing down his fall enough to save his life. (WM)

* * *

"Stress and pain thus become
potentially valuable portals
and motivations through
which to enter the
practice."

Coming
to Our enses,
Jon Kabat-Zinn

Although he survived, Oliver's landing was so severe that he spent the next few weeks in a coma. Will, Mysteria, and Edgar rested quietly within Oliver's physical body during this time, as it healed from the trauma.

After weeks had passed, it became time for Oliver to reclaim his conscious state of being. Both Will and Mysteria knew that this time would be challenging for him and that he and Edgar would need them more than ever. (WM) The doctors entered the room to examine Oliver and found him moaning and slowly becoming conscious. Upon waking and trying to move, Oliver quickly realized he was immobile and could not feel anything from his neck down. Will and Mysteria went into overdrive trying to comfort Oliver as he wept end-lessly. (WM)

Paralysis had taken hold of Oliver's body and this fate was more than Edgar could handle. Oliver asked himself, "How will the world treat me now that I'm quadriplegic? My parents?" (WM)

"Death would be easier," thought Edgar. Will and Mysteria tried to comfort Edgar as Oliver was fitted for a wheelchair. "I can't do this!" exclaimed Edgar. "I can't live this way." Will and Mysteria began to make their presence more known by increasing their auditory sound, trying to overshadow Edgar's insistent fear. (WM) Will expanded sweetly as Mysteria softened, trying to comfort and settle Oliver's anxiety. Oliver could feel the conflicted emotions stirring within. (WM)

His parents visited him frequently and briefly. Oliver could sense their discomfort, how lost they felt trying to meet his current needs. It made him wonder if they had dismissed their own vulnerability long ago and found themselves powerless in relation to their own children. Maybe it was easier and more rewarding for them to assist strangers than their own loved ones. Or could it be that strangers may have appreciated them more?

A sadness flooded Oliver as he recognized some painful truths. He realized he could no longer run away from his feelings, busy himself with life's many to-dos, or escape from the reality of his situation. His immobility forced him to face some difficult feelings. His doctor repeatedly sent the hospital's yoga teacher, Veronica, to his room to move his limbs around, but Edgar would yell at her, saying, "What's the point? I can't feel them—leave me alone."

One day, Veronica came to visit and found Oliver sleeping. She could see for the first time how peaceful he could actually be. She decided to record this peacefulness, the sound of Will and Mysteria symphonically rising and falling as he rested. She then played the recording over the room's sound system. Upon waking, Oliver was greeted with the sound of his own breath, amplified throughout the room with penetrating strength and power. (WM) It was so rhythmic and peaceful that he found it hard to believe it was just his inhale and exhale. (WM) Miraculously, he began to feel alive again! (WM)

Now curious about his breath, Oliver strived to do breathing exercises daily, as Veronica had instructed. Will and Mysteria loved this new attention from Oliver, and Veronica knew this practice would bring Oliver peace as he tried to deal with the reality of his new life. (WM) She told Oliver, "In Sanskrit, the word *asana* means 'to sit with what is.' When we are able to accept what life brings us and find peace within that acceptance, we become liberated. True acceptance, ironically, can make space for unimaginable (beyond your wildest dreams) changes, making it the most rewarding posture in yoga. Oliver, if you can master this great *asana*, there's no need to master the physical ones." (WM)

* * *

Some months later, after scattered visits from family and friends, sporadic angry moments, and various life disappointments, a mysterious calm began to enter Oliver's being. (WM) Veronica taught him Ujjayi breathing, a technique of breathing in and out through the nose, allowing Will and Mysteria to draw through the back of the throat for a powerful sound and vibration. (WM)

Each time he paused to recognize his breath, he found himself absorbed into its sound, its warmth, and its comfort. (WM) He noticed how his breath settled the restless thoughts that Edgar churned out and brought Oliver further away from his illusions and fears. (WM) Oliver began to find great comfort and companionship in his breath; Will and Mysteria became like new best friends he could count on. (WM) He began to practice

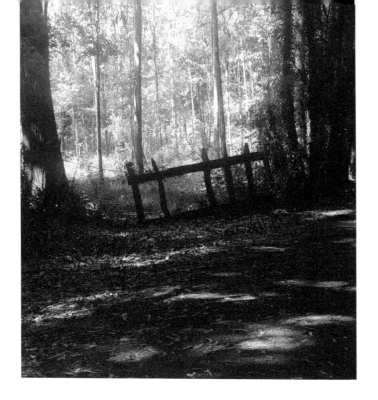

being in their presence both day and night, realizing that even in his frequent solitary moments he was never really alone. For his lungs, Veronica shared, are his wings turned inward, and he can now soar from the inside, expanding far and wide. (WM)

This continuous acknowledgment of Will and Mysteria prompted Oliver's presence to grow and a frequently neglected indweller in his chest named Haven began to make itself known. Expanding with expressive joy from the inside, Oliver felt compelled to spread these feelings to his outside world. He soon found himself mentoring the young orphaned children of Galore teaching them about nature, helping them to recognize their own true nature. (WM)

* * *

Will & Mysteria were magically emphasizing the NOW when to his elated surprise, Oliver was given a new job as the first energy professor at Galore University. This position would allow him and Edgar to explore new pathways for developing renewable energy sources. One evening, he was reading about his new position, when a light streamed through the window and cast an orange-red glow across his body. He motored his wheelchair close to the window, and he could see the setting sun casting a stunning light on the rising harvest moon. (WM) Immediately, he felt a radiant and calming presence. Will and Mysteria began to expand, and Oliver began to smile; they recognized the presence of RaLuna. They were awed by this second visit. (WM)

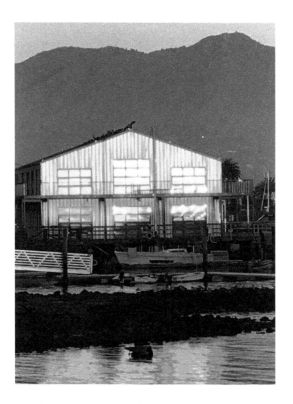

RaLuna's presence was so profound it immediately softened Edgar's grip on Oliver's mind. At the same moment the hair on Oliver's arms began to rise. Oliver looked down in utter disbelief. The sight and the sensation were overwhelming. Tears began to stream down his face. (WM) He could feel his arms for the first time since the accident. He joyously wept as he felt Will and Mysteria moving through all his limbs. (WM) His gaze returned to the sunset, and he heard a voice whisper,

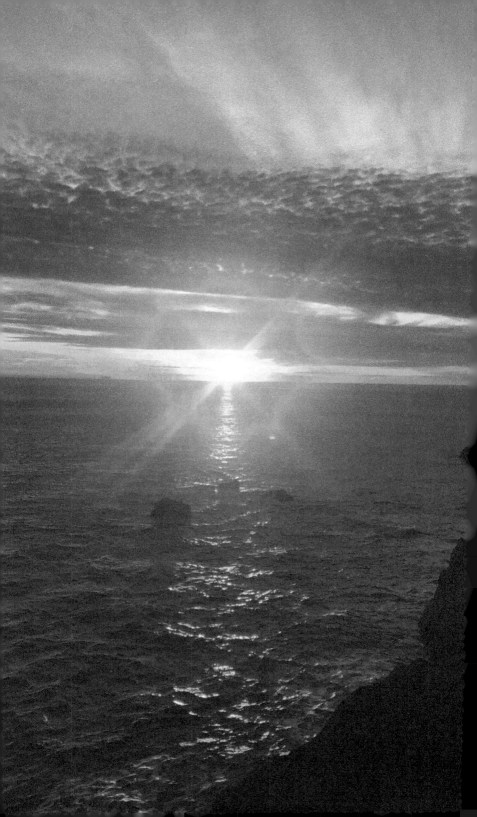

"By befriending your loving spirit within, you will never be without." (WM)

With that, the sun set, leaving a blinding blue-green flash.

* * *

"Your breathing can be an exquisite guide towards a way of being
that is transformative not only for
yourself but for all those that come
into contact with you"

The Breathing Book,
Donna Farhi

DISCUSSION QUESTIONS

Can you relate to Will and if so, how?

Can you relate to Mysteria and if so, how?

Can you relate to Edgar and if so, how?

Mysteria operates by releasing old cellular memory, what does this mean to you and your ability to heal yourself?

When is Edgar useful in our lives; why does he need to be alive and well in our human framework?

Does RaLuna show up in your life, if so, how?

How has your awareness of your breath changed your life or your health?

Is Haven active and in service within you, if so, how?

Please Note: Will & Mysteria was originally meant to be an illustrated adult children's book, however, spirit intervened and most of the photos in this book were compliments of nature here in my hometown and my personal iphone. (all rights reserved) Please enjoy capturing RaLuna's energy in most of the photographs that include the sun. Thank You, Magical Universe!

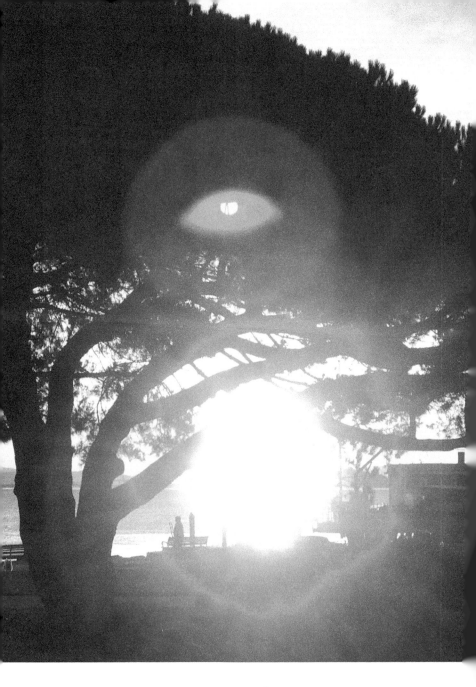

Third Eye Orb of the SUN

AFTERWORD

Why did I write this story? Yoga is an internal process. There are many amazing "how to" books in the market place that delve into the yoga *asanas*, or the Sanskrit literature. I have been so blessed over the years to learn and reference from these brilliant books as well as the incredible live masters I've had the privilege to study with, to include Sarah Powers, Tias Little (Breath Master) and Jack Kornfield to name just a few. In this book, I wanted to see if an adventuresome story could elicit the reader's feelings, requesting presence and providing an opportunity for reflection. Could we as a culture return to myths and parables, the ancient way our spiritual teachers use to teach us (Jack Kornfield and Sarah Powers still do), by enrolling the reader, their imagination and simply giving them the opportunity to see themselves within the story? Will and Mysteria's intention is to ignite our inner observatory skills while engaging the mind and body to work together.

I also had my own ego structures to work out and come to terms with; the places inside me that we're both ambitious and deeply terrified to succeed. Who of us has not at some point in our lives been stuck in ego paralysis, analyzing the crap out of our lives and unable to move or evolve anywhere? Will & Mysteria was originally written in 2006, and it took until 2018 for me to summon the courage to put this story out in the world.

On a more intimate level, it has also been my ongoing process and journey for the past 30 plus years, to make sense of the many confused parts inside myself. I grew up courageous but also very afraid; vigilant and yet unaware; needing to trust but often struggling to truly trust; wanting deeply to be loved while often forgetting to love myself.

I took my mother by complete surprise: she thought she was having her last baby of four, but days before giving birth, she learned of me, stuffed behind my twin brother. The thought of five kids under the age of six threw her into overwhelm. We started off on the wrong foot and traveled a difficult emotional road. Feeling estranged at times within my family, I found myself acting out in erratic ways growing up, unconsciously grasping for attention.

My spiritual journey began upon my first Saturn Return (twenty-nine years old) with me exploring Shamanism. I was drawn to nature, and I learned early on "the earth is our alter and everything is sacred." However my Shaman at the time, Brant Secunda, quickly showed me how I kept leaving my body due to early trauma and how I needed to master staying embodied if I was ever going to help anyone. I was soon dreaming my yoga world into existence.

In the early stages of my yoga practice, as self-aware-ness was unfolding, the sting of my perceived inadequacies were piercing, heart-wrenching, and skin erupting.

These imagined but sometime real deficiencies provoked great anxiety as I decided on a career as a public yoga teacher—a position in which you can't hide from your journey, and your struggles seep into your practice and your life no matter what. Although it was a profound privilege to share what I was learning with my students, it was often from these inspired places as well as the emotional difficulties that we yoga teachers help others see their journey and our collective humanness. My inner parts soon became my best friends as I had nowhere else to turn. I could not afford ongoing therapy nor could I continue to endlessly talk about my struggles with my friends. It needed to be transformed with time, attention, and my embodied yoga practice.

Fending for myself growing up, I learned how to have a relationship with these various internal parts of me. After many years of seeking, I finally got in contact with the ringleader, my RaLuna. Today, these internal conversations are many and endless as I try to construct each day in the likeness of "being," with grace and understanding first for myself and then for others.

My mother and I have healed so much between us over the past fifteen years, by acknowledging some painful truths, seeing our humanness and exercising acceptance. I saw how I was constantly wishing life to be other than what it was, people to be other than who they were. Learning to truly accept life as it is has been my redemption. Today, my mother truly lives in my heart; my early sadness and pain have all but disappeared. I'm not sure I would have ever let go of my juvenile reactions without Will and Mysteria consciously awakening me through the practice of yoga and meditation. They are my closest and dearest tenants now. (On a more fun note, my mother went on to have one more child after my twin and I that she laughingly refers to as her "mint julep baby" the Kentucky Derby surprise.)

* * *

The actual story of Will and Mysteria sprang from a yoga and kayaking trip I took to the island of Crete in 2005. I went with a company out of my hometown of Chicago called Northwest Passage. We would kayak from coastal town to coastal town, often along the water's edge, taking in the beautiful vistas. We happened upon a little town that was known for its delicious Greek food and one innkeeper's private residence in a cove down the coast. Our first day there, we ventured out kayaking towards this private home. Upon arriving at their private property, we saw that the grounds were marked with many large boulders and lots of little rocks displayed everywhere. It was hardly our anticipated sandy beach.

The house was locked and all but boarded up, and the only redeeming aspect was the homemade ladder that climbed up the boarding wall of the cove. This ladder had been constructed by the family's son for his entertainment and was made of simple yet sturdy wire and horizontal wood slats. It was bolted down and scaled the uneven cliff wall, going straight up some sixty plus feet. Simply looking up to the top made my neck ache! Ryan, one of our free-spirited guides from Northwest Passage, decided he would ascend this wall and grab a glimpse of the vista above. He had brought other groups here before, and because his last ascent had been successful, he didn't hesitate to give it another go. We held our breath as we watched him climb, little pieces of earth falling down on us as we shrieked in discomfort. Ryan managed to reach the top and waved to us tiny ants below.

After descending back down, Ryan asked if anyone else would like to try going up. He mentioned that no woman had ever reached the top. I was both intrigued by the idea of climbing to the top and terrified by the many rocks below.

My Edgar (though I hadn't yet assigned that name) was now shifting crazily inside. My self-esteem was a tad low, and my need to feel accomplished and be seen quite high! Nervously, and with limbs rattling, I began my ascent.

About a third of the way up, looking down was no longer an option, real fear began to kick in, and a voice inside was now taking over. It was my breath. I began to really hear it, and it soon became the impetus by which I moved my limbs from one slat to the next. Every step I took was with an audible inhale and exhale. It became my only focus. I was as present as I had ever been. My inhale and my exhale settled my mind and allowed me to focus on the slats that my feet dug into so as not to slip. I'll never forget how my inhales and exhales—which I later named Will and Mysteria—nurtured me, calmed me, and allowed me to be the first woman ever to scale this ladder to the top!

We returned that night to the family's inn for dinner, and I was truly celebrated by the people of the small town. Many came over and congratulated me. It was my Edgar that led me to this dangerous challenge, but it was Will and Mysteria that allowed me to succeed! Looking back, it was definitely one of the stupider things I've done in this lifetime—and yet one of the wisest, as I now have two magnificent and trustworthy friends for life, Will and Mysteria. (WM)

For more information about the author, her breath and meditation workshops, speaking engagements or the books availability please email: info@willandmysteria.com

BREATH EXERCISES

Please enjoy these simple and yet invigorating **breath exercises** that are designed to calm the central nervous system, quiet down the mind from the busy mental chatter, and release any tension from the body so it can relax.

Calming Breath Meditation

3-5 minutes; can be done anytime during the day!

Bring yourself to a seated position, ideally on a yoga block or cushion so your hips are raised a bit and your ankles cross on the floor before you. This can also be done in a straight-backed chair with sit bones firmly on seat, back upright, feet planted on the floor.

Begin by closing the mouth and drawing breath in slowly through the back of the throat and the nose as you feel your belly and your lungs beginning to fill, shoulders rolling back a bit. Once full, transition into an exhale as your eyes begin to close (Acquire these MP3 meditations for free by emailing info@willandmysteria.com). Feel your vertebrae stack one on top of the other, your sit bones grounding and your shoulders relaxing.

Draw breath in slowly. This time after you fill up with breath, transition to the exhale by feeling your muscles relax to the bone, your blood flowing through your veins, your stomach soften, your jaw and eye sockets relaxing.

Drawing breath in again, bring this inhale into the space between the brain and the skull, shrinking the brain a bit. As you exhale feel the release of any tension, anxiety, or nervousness; the jaw relaxing again and the back of the eye sockets opening. Drawing breath in again slowly bring this expansiveness into the frontal lobe and the back of the head, imagine an open book before you with lots of words, displaying all your mental constructs, busyness of the mind, chatter, or worries. Now as you exhale, imagine them just fall away like words falling off a page until you see a blank page before you in your mind's eye. Allow your mind to become neutral and present, looking inward at a blank page, simply observing the rise and fall of your breath through the body for another minute.

To finish, bring the hands to prayer *mudra* at the heart center, bow your head, and listen for a moment into your heart; see if it has any wisdom or insight for you. Then take a nice breath in, and exhale, bowing in Namaste.

"May I meet this breath as a friend"
—Sylvia Boorstein, author
Pay Attention for Goodness Sake

Breath Of Fire - Ego Eradicator

This breath work is referred to by different names depending on the yoga tradition in which you are working. Its formal name is Kalapalabhati otherwise known as clearing breath or breath of fire. In the Kundalini tradition it is utilized frequently for the internal cleansing process. For our purposes here we will introduce the eagle pose also known as "Ego Eradicator". It is best done first thing in the morning or late afternoon. It is a very energizing posture that builds your aura, detoxifies the body, gives clarity of mind, supports digestion and will replenish your energy while increasing your radiance.

Begin by sitting up tall either on a cushion on the floor or in a straight back chair with the soles of the feet on the floor. Lift hands and curl the four fingers inward having the finger pads touch the palm while stretching the thumbs as far away as you can from your curled fingers. Point thumbs at each other as you raise arms above head at sixty degrees apart for short quick breaths. If you have never done this type of breathing please open your mouth and stick your tongue out. Then begin to pant like a dog until you can feel your stomach move in and out quickly. Close your mouth and push this same breath through your nose quickly and rhythmically.

Allow your shoulders to soften as your heart floats upwards. Look inward at your third eye.

This breath should be done for a minimum of one minute and upwards of three minutes to see real results on a daily basis. When you've completed 1–3 minutes, you will take a slow inhale and draw the thumbs towards each other to touch above your head, open the curled fingers up to the heavens holding the breath for a count of five and releasing the arms as you exhale. Sit quietly for another 1–2 minutes feeling the body continue to cleanse and purify your system. Our Edgar or our "Ego" can be relentless and irritating, and it's important we keep clearing our energy especially around the third chakra (solar plexus) so we can lead with love and intelligence.

Please visit my website to download a free MP3 of these breathing meditations and a bonus one that is not displayed here. Enjoy your new freedom!

"Breath" by Kabir

Are you looking for me?
I am in the next seat.
My shoulder is against yours.
You will not find me in the stupas,
Not in the Indian shrine rooms,
Nor in synagogues,
Nor in cathedrals,
Nor in masses,
Nor kirtans,
Not in legs winding around your own neck,
Nor in eating nothing but vegetables.

When you really look for me,
You will feel me instantly –
You will find me in the tiniest house of time.
Kabir says: Students, tell me, what is God?
He is the breath inside the breath."
—Kabir

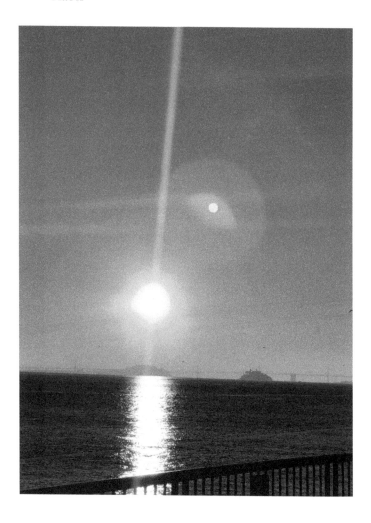

Truth Is Crazier Than Fiction

Magic abounds: just weeks before my final proof of this book a new friend of mine named Tracey (who did not know anything about me publishing a book) happened to share with me a gentleman she met at a Dr. Joe Dispenza meet up in San Leandro, California. She explained his body has quadriplegia and he is having remarkable healing from his recent breath work, meditation, light and sound therapies. I had the fortunate opportunity to meet Chris and discuss his personal story and my book Will & Mysteria. He marvels at the incredible sensations and energy he's moving with his attention on his inner being!

Meet Chris and please reach out to learn about his journey and inspiring platform at: www.ChrisFinn.com

> "Bravo to Christa for bringing to light in such a unique and highly personable way (especially for me living with quadriplegia) the simple things that are good to focus on that makes such a huge difference in our lives!"
>
> Chris Finn

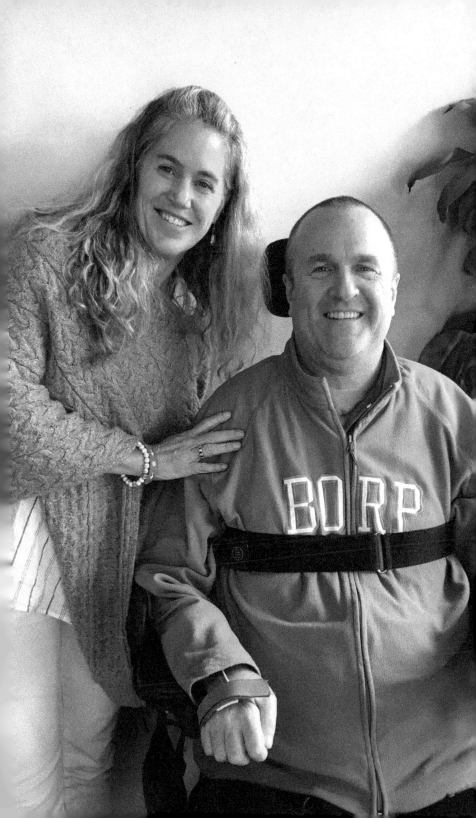

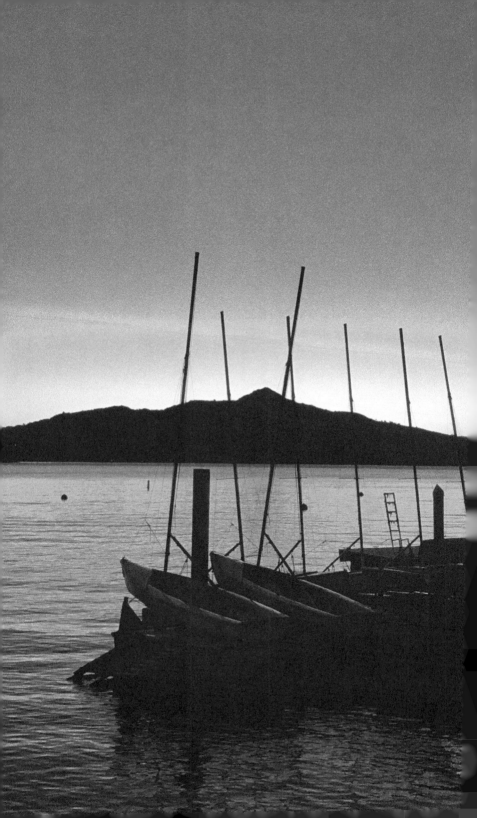

BUY_{ME}
READ_{ME}
&
GIFT_{ME}

PRINT YOUR NAME – CITY – STATE
& Pass it ON!

Once 5-10 people have read *Will & Mysteria*, please post a picture of their names (or just their city and state) on social media for the original purchaser of the book.

SHARING OUR WEALTH…IMPROVING
OUR HEALTH!

CPSIA information can be obtained
at www.ICGtesting.com
Printed in the USA
BVHW091942131019
561005BV00001B/1/P